Simplified Solution Approach
To OSTEOARTHRITIS

Revitalize Your Body, Rediscover Freedom:
Break Free from Joint Discomfort with
Proven Strategies for Lasting Relief

Dr QUENTIN GLYN

Table Of Contents

CHAPTER ONE
Osteoarthritis

Millions of individuals worldwide suffer from osteoarthritis (OA), a degenerative joint condition that causes pain, stiffness, and decreased mobility. Osteoarthritis is one of the main causes of disability and a major public health concern. The goal of this book is to provide a straightforward method for managing and lessening the effects of osteoarthritis on people and communities.

A Synopsis Of Osteoarthritis:

The destruction of cartilage in joints, which causes pain, swelling, and alterations in the bone, is the hallmark of osteoarthritis. Even though it often affects the hands, spine, knees, and hips, it may affect every joint in the body. Due to its degenerative nature, osteoarthritis (OA) is a chronic illness that is often linked to obesity, joint traumas, and age. Osteoarthritis is quite common, however, it has no known cure. The main goals of therapy are to control symptoms and enhance the quality of life for individuals who have the condition.

The Need To Treat Osteoarthritis:

Osteoarthritis affects people widely and has a significant financial effect on healthcare systems. The long-term discomfort and limited movement linked to osteoarthritis (OA) can result in a lower standard of living, higher medical expenses, and a substantial financial strain. We hope to equip people with the information and resources they need to actively manage their condition, lessen symptoms, and improve their general well-being by creating a simplified solution approach.

The Objective Of The Book:

This book's main goal is to demystify osteoarthritis and give readers doable, approachable strategies for successfully managing the ailment. We intend to close the knowledge gap between complicated medical information and common sense tactics people can use to lessen the effects of osteoarthritis on their daily lives by providing a simplified approach.

The causes, symptoms, risk factors, and treatments available for osteoarthritis are just a few of the many topics covered in this book. Even though we make every effort to offer thorough information, it's critical to recognize the limitations that come with oversimplifying a complicated medical condition. People are encouraged to seek personalized medical advice from healthcare professionals rather than relying solely on this book.

A Roadmap Leading To The Resolution:

The book is designed to walk readers through a methodical approach to osteoarthritis management. It starts with a thorough analysis of the illness and moves on to discuss realistic methods for managing it over the long term, changing one's lifestyle, and relieving symptoms. Every chapter expands on the one before it, giving readers a clear and easy path to follow.

In conclusion, "Simplified Solution Approach to Osteoarthritis" strives to equip people with the information and resources required to manage the problems offered by osteoarthritis. This book aims to increase the accessibility and achievableness of osteoarthritis management for a larger range of readers by offering a clear road map and useful strategies.

CHAPTER TWO

Understanding Osteoarthritis

Definition And Causes:

Osteoarthritis (OA) is a degenerative joint disease that predominantly affects the articular cartilage, the protective tissue surrounding the ends of bones in a joint. It is the most prevalent kind of arthritis, and its frequency rises with age. OA may develop in any joint, although it most typically affects the knees, hips, hands, and spine.

The fundamental cause of osteoarthritis is the degradation of cartilage. Cartilage is a hard, rubbery layer that covers the ends of bones in normal joints and functions as a cushion between bones. Over time, the cartilage might wear away, causing discomfort, edema, and limited joint mobility. The specific etiology of cartilage degradation in OA is complicated and may involve a mix of genetic, environmental, and mechanical factors.

Risk Factors:

1. Age: The risk of osteoarthritis grows with age, as the wear and strain on joints build over time.

2. Gender: Osteoarthritis is more common in women than in males, particularly after the age of 50.

3. Genetics: OA is predisposed to by genetics. You can be more vulnerable if any of your parents or siblings have OA.

4. Joint Overuse or Injury: Overuse of joints in certain jobs or activities, as well as past joint traumas, may all lead to the development of osteoarthritis (OA).

5. Obesity: Carrying too much weight around strains weight-bearing joints including the knees and hips, increasing the risk of osteoarthritis (OA).

6. Joint malalignment: Osteoarthritis may result from abnormal joint structure or malalignment, which can cause uneven wear on the joint surfaces.

When a joint develops osteoarthritis, it experiences many structural changes.

1. Cartilage Degeneration: The bone underneath is exposed when the articular cartilage thins and/or wears away completely.

2. Bone Changes: At the joint's margins, bone spurs, or osteophytes, may form, exacerbating discomfort and restricting range of motion.

3. Inflammation of the Synovial Membrane: The synovial membrane, which lubricates joints and lines their capsules, may become inflamed.

4. Ligament Changes: Bone remodeling and ligament thickening are possible outcomes.

Typical Symptoms:

1. Discomfort: Prolonged joint discomfort that usually gets better at rest and becomes worse when you move.

2. Stiffness: Stiffness in the joints, particularly after periods of inactivity, such as waking up in the morning.

3. Swelling: Inflammatory swelling around the afflicted joint.

4. Reduced Range of Motion: The joint's inability to move through its whole range of motion.

5. Joint Instability: A sensation of giving way or instability in the joints.

Methods Of Diagnosis:

1. Medical History and Physical Examination: Osteoarthritis may be diagnosed with the use of a thorough medical history and a physical examination.

2. Imaging Research:

• X-rays: To evaluate cartilage loss, bone spurs, and joint injury.

• Magnetic Resonance Imaging (MRI): Offers fine-grained pictures of soft tissues, such as ligaments and cartilage.

3. Blood Tests: Certain tests may help rule out other kinds of arthritis, but there isn't a particular blood test for osteoarthritis.

4. Joint Fluid Analysis: To rule out other possible causes and discover inflammation, synovial fluid from the afflicted joint may be removed and examined.

5. Arthroscopy: To directly see the joint and determine the degree of injury, a surgeon may sometimes use an arthroscope, a tiny tube equipped with a camera.

For an easier way to manage osteoarthritis, it is essential to comprehend the causes, risk factors, architecture of afflicted joints, prevalent symptoms, and diagnostic techniques. Implementing techniques to reduce symptoms and enhance the quality of life for people with OA may be aided by early diagnosis and management.

CHAPTER THREE

Osteoarthritis's Effect On Everyday Life

Osteoarthritis's Consequence Scheduled Daily Time:

Physical Limitations: A person's everyday functioning and physical capacities are greatly impacted by osteoarthritis (OA). Joint cartilage gradually deteriorates, resulting in discomfort, stiffness, and a restricted range of motion. Even ordinary tasks like walking, climbing stairs, and even gripping items become difficult. These physical restrictions might make a person less independent and more dependent on outside help or assistive technology.

Emotional Impact: Managing chronic pain is a common aspect of living with osteoarthritis, and this may have a significant emotional impact. Anxiety and despair may be exacerbated by ongoing pain and the annoyance of being unable to carry out daily tasks. The effect on mental health is not exclusive to the person affected; family members and caregivers may also be emotionally strained as a result of seeing the challenges.

Social Repercussions: Social interactions and activities may be hampered by osteoarthritis. Due to the condition's physical restrictions, social interaction may be less frequent, which might result in feelings of loneliness and isolation. People with OA may find it difficult to maintain an active social life or go on social excursions when their mobility declines, which might have an impact on their general well-being.

Economic Burden: Osteoarthritis has a complex financial effect. Expenses for prescription drugs, surgeries, and medical care are considered direct expenditures. Indirect expenses are also a part of productivity losses brought on by subpar job output or lost workdays. The cost burden may also be increased by the need for assistive technology, house changes, and adjustments to transportation. Osteoarthritis may have significant long-term cost effects on people as well as healthcare systems since it is often a chronic ailment.

Quality of Life: The general quality of life is significantly impacted by osteoarthritis. A lowered feeling of well-being may result from the interaction of social restraints, mental suffering, and physical limits. A person's social connections, mental and emotional stability, physical health, and capacity for meaningful activity are just a few of the elements that make up their overall quality of life. Each of these elements may be compromised by osteoarthritis, which can have an impact on how happy and satisfied a person feels with their life.

Simplified Method Of Solving:

Pain management: It's essential to put into practice efficient pain management techniques.

A mix of physical therapy, medication, and lifestyle changes may be used to achieve this. Exercise, weight control, and joint protection measures are examples of non-pharmacological strategies that are essential for reducing pain and preserving joint function.

Emotional Support: It's important to acknowledge and deal with the emotional effects of osteoarthritis. Giving people access to therapy, support groups, and mental health services may help them deal with the psychological difficulties brought on by physical limits and chronic pain. It's also advantageous to include family members in the support system.

Encouraging social inclusion is essential to reducing the negative social effects of osteoarthritis. Enhancing social participation may be achieved via developing accessible venues, planning activities specifically for those with restricted mobility, and cultivating a supportive community. Fostering transparent dialogue and comprehension among colleagues may also aid in creating a more welcoming social atmosphere.

Workplace Accommodations: One way to alleviate the financial strain is to provide accommodations for those with osteoarthritis in the workplace. Reducing economic hardship and productivity losses, flexible work hours, ergonomic changes, and disability accommodations may help people stay in or return to the workforce.

Holistic Approach to Healthcare: A holistic approach to healthcare takes into account all of the many aspects of a person's life that are impacted by osteoarthritis. This includes social assistance, rehabilitation, and all-encompassing medical treatment. Working together, healthcare providers, caregivers, and community services may provide a more comprehensive and successful strategy for controlling osteoarthritis's effects on day-to-day functioning.

In conclusion, treating the physical, emotional, social, and economic facets of osteoarthritis is necessary for a thorough and straightforward approach to treatment.

People with osteoarthritis may improve their overall quality of life and well-being by putting into practice pain management, emotional support, social inclusion, employment adjustments, and holistic healthcare initiatives.

CHAPTER FOUR
Current Methods Of Treatment

The degenerative joint condition known as osteoarthritis (OA) is characterized by the deterioration of both the underlying bone and cartilage. Although osteoarthritis is a chronic illness for which there is no known cure, there are a number of treatment options that try to control symptoms and enhance the quality of life for those who have it.

Drugs:

Pain Relievers (Analgesics): Ibuprofen and naproxen, two nonsteroidal anti-inflammatory medications (NSAIDs), are often used to treat pain and decrease inflammation.

Acetaminophen is often suggested as a pain reliever, particularly for those who are unable to use NSAIDs because of gastrointestinal problems or other contraindications.

Topical medications: To relieve pain locally, creams, patches, or gels containing capsaicin or NSAIDs may be administered directly to the injured joint.

Physical Medicine:

Exercise Programs: Tailor-made workout plans that include flexibility, strength, and cardio activities may help relieve pain and enhance joint function.

Manual Therapy: Physical therapists may use methods like massage and joint manipulation to increase joint mobility and decrease stiffness.

Assistive Devices: To lessen joint stress and increase stability, braces, canes, or other supporting devices may be advised.

Surgical Procedures:

Joint Replacement Surgery: When all other therapies have failed and the condition is severe, joint replacement surgery may be an option. This entails substituting a prosthetic joint—usually in the hip or knee—for the injured one.

Arthroscopy: A minimally invasive treatment that involves assessing and fixing joint injury by inserting a tiny tube equipped with a camera.

Osteotomy: A surgical treatment in which the afflicted joint is relieved of pressure by reshaping the bones.

Modifications In Lifestyle:

Weight control: Keeping a healthy weight lessens the strain on the knees and hips, two joints that carry a lot of weight.

Joint protection: Using assistive technology and avoiding too repetitive motions are two methods to protect joints throughout everyday tasks.

Balanced Diet: Eating a healthy, vitamin- and mineral-rich diet promotes joint health in general.

Constraints On Current Therapies:

Symptomatic Relief: Rather than treating the underlying cause of osteoarthritis, the majority of current therapies concentrate on controlling symptoms. As a result, it becomes a chronic illness that needs constant care.

Medications' adverse effects include gastrointestinal distress, cardiovascular difficulties, and other negative effects that might arise with long-term use of NSAIDs and other painkillers.

Limited Effectiveness in Disease Modification: Current therapies are unable to significantly stimulate cartilage repair or delay the advancement of osteoarthritis.

The hazard and expense of surgery are two things that come with the procedure, even if some people find it to be successful. Long recovery times might also have an adverse effect on the patient's quality of life.

In conclusion, while current treatment modalities help people with osteoarthritis function better and relieve their symptoms, they are not always effective in treating the underlying cause of the condition or bringing about long-term change. Innovative treatments and interventions are still being investigated in order to provide people with osteoarthritis with more complete and efficient care.

CHAPTER FIVE

The Framework For Simplified Solutions

Osteoarthritis (OA) is a common degenerative joint disease that causes pain, stiffness, and impaired joint function due to cartilage degradation. A thorough and simple solution structure is needed to handle the intricacies of open access. This paradigm emphasizes a patient-centered approach, incorporates traditional and alternative treatments, and creates personalized treatment regimens.

A Comprehensive Approach To Osteoarthritis:

a. Grasping the Big Picture:

Realizing that OA is a multifactorial condition including genes, lifestyle, and general health rather than just being a localized joint problem.

Stressing the significance of treating the underlying causes and contributing variables in addition to the symptoms.

b. All-encompassing Evaluation:

Completing a comprehensive assessment of the patient's lifestyle, mental health, and medical background.

Working together with a diverse group of medical experts, such as physiotherapists, dietitians, rheumatologists, and mental health specialists.

Combining Traditional And Alternative Medical Treatments:

a. Traditional Therapies:

Using strategies that are supported by science, such as physical therapy, NSAIDs, and painkillers.

investigating surgical options, such as joint replacement procedures, when they are required.

b. Alternative Medical Interventions:

Combining alternative methods to relieve pain and increase joint flexibility, such as massage therapy, yoga, and acupuncture.

investigating the advantages of dietary supplements and nutraceuticals, such as chondroitin and glucosamine, to promote joint health.

Patient-First Healthcare:

a. Patient Empowerment:

Encouraging informed consent and collaborative decision-making in order to promote active involvement in their treatment programs.

Promoting candid dialogue to meet the needs, preferences, and therapeutic objectives of the patient.

b. Tailored Care:

Realizing that every patient's experience with OA is different and needs tailored care.

adjusting therapies according to the patient's general health, lifestyle, and symptom intensity.

Tailored Treatment Programs:

a. Multimodal Methods:

Creating all-encompassing treatment programs that include medical, physical, and psychological therapies.

Modifying treatment plans in light of the disease's course and each patient's reaction to a given course of therapy.

b. Extended-Term Administration:

putting long-term management concepts into practice with an emphasis on exercise routines, lifestyle changes, and continuing support.

evaluating and modifying the treatment plan on a regular basis to take into account changes in the patient's condition and new therapeutic possibilities.

Osteoarthritis may be simplified using a paradigm that takes a patient-centered approach, taking into account their overall health. Healthcare practitioners may improve the efficacy of OA management by combining traditional and alternative treatments, emphasizing patient-centric care, and creating customized treatment programs. In addition to treating the symptoms, this method gives patients the confidence to take an active role in their health, which promotes an all-encompassing and long-lasting approach to osteoarthritis treatment.

CHAPTER SIX
Osteoarthritis Dietary Strategies

Osteoarthritis is a degenerative joint condition that causes pain and stiffness in the afflicted joints due to the deterioration of cartilage. Osteoarthritis has no known treatment, although nutritional approaches are vital for controlling symptoms and enhancing joint health in general.

Nutrition's Significance:

Since nutrition has a direct impact on the health of the joints and surrounding tissues, it is essential for controlling osteoarthritis.

Maintaining a healthy weight eases the strain on weight-bearing joints such as the hips and knees when a person eats a well-balanced and nutrient-rich diet. Important elements that assist cartilage preservation and repair are also provided by a healthy diet.

Foods That Reduce Inflammation:

One important element in the development of osteoarthritis is inflammation. Anti-inflammatory foods may help reduce inflammation and halt the progression of the disease. Foods that reduce inflammation include:

1. Fatty Fish: Packed with omega-3 fatty acids, fish with anti-inflammatory qualities that help relieve joint pain include salmon, mackerel, and sardines.

2. Vibrant Fruits and Vegetables: Rich in anti-inflammatory and antioxidant properties including berries, cherries, and dark greens.

3. Nuts and Seeds: Rich in omega-3 fatty acids and offering anti-inflammatory properties including almonds, walnuts, flaxseeds, and chia seeds.

4. Turmeric and Ginger: These spices have strong anti-inflammatory properties due to the contents of curcumin and gingerol, respectively.

5. Extra virgin olive oil: Packed with antioxidants and monounsaturated fats, this oil has anti-inflammatory properties.

Vitamins & Supplements:

Certain vitamins and supplements help improve joint health and lessen osteoarthritis symptoms. See a medical expert before incorporating supplements into your regimen. Among the supplements that are often advised are:

1. Natural substances present in cartilage are glucosamine and chondroitin. Supplements may aid with joint function improvement and pain reduction.

2.Omega-3 Fatty Acids: Supplementing with fish oil may give you more omega-3s to help reduce inflammation.

3. Vitamin D: Important for strong bones, vitamin D aids in the absorption of calcium and may slow the development of osteoarthritis.

4. Calcium: A healthy diet rich in calcium is essential for strong bones and the prevention of osteoporosis, which may aggravate joint problems.

Drinking Plenty Of Water:

Drinking enough water is crucial for healthy joints. Water facilitates smoother movement and lowers friction by lubricating joints. Dehydration may aggravate symptoms and be a contributing factor to stiff joints. Make it a point to stay hydrated throughout the day by drinking enough water.

Recipes And Diet Plans:

1. The Mediterranean Diet

• Places a focus on entire grains, fruits, vegetables, and healthy fats.

• Contains modest quantities of lean protein from chicken and fish.

Utilizes olive oil as the main fat source.

2. Smoothie for Inflammation Relief:

• For a wholesome and anti-inflammatory smoothie, blend spinach, berries, banana, Greek yogurt, and a teaspoon of turmeric together.

3. Salad with Salmon:

• Seared salmon with cherry tomatoes, cucumbers, and a drizzle of olive oil served over a bed of mixed greens.

4. Bowl of Quinoa:

• Quinoa combined with chickpeas, sautéed veggies, and a dash of almonds to provide more omega-3 fatty acids.

5. Ginger-Turmeric Tea:

To make a calming and anti-inflammatory tea, combine turmeric, ginger, and a small amount of honey.

To sum up, implementing a well-rounded diet that prioritizes anti-inflammatory foods, in addition to taking the right supplements and being hydrated, may prove to be a successful approach in the management of osteoarthritis.

In order to customize these dietary plans to your unique requirements and medical condition, always seek the advice of a qualified nutritionist or healthcare provider.

CHAPTER SEVEN
Physical Activity And Recovery

Osteoarthritis (OA) is a common degenerative joint disease that causes pain, stiffness, and limited range of motion due to the destruction of cartilage in the joints. Although there isn't a cure for osteoarthritis, joint function may be improved, symptoms can be managed, and general well-being can be increased with exercise and rehabilitation.

Customized Fitness Plans:
Customized Evaluation:

A comprehensive evaluation by a medical expert or physical therapist is essential prior to starting any kind of fitness program. This aids in determining certain joint restrictions, muscle deficiencies, and personal objectives.

Exercise for the Heart:

It's common advice to engage in low-impact aerobic activities like cycling, swimming, or walking. By improving cardiovascular health, these exercises save the joints from undue strain.

Exercises Targeting the Joints:

Exercises must be specifically designed to target the joints that osteoarthritis affects. Leg raises, quadriceps strengthening, and knee extensions are a few examples of knee workouts.

Minimal-Impact Exercises:

Exercise in the Water:

Activities that include water, like swimming or water aerobics, are great choices for those who have osteoarthritis. Water's buoyancy provides resistance for strength training while lessening the strain on joints.

Cycling:

A low-impact workout that helps increase joint flexibility and range of motion is riding a stationary or normal bike. It's particularly helpful for those who have osteoarthritis in their hips or knees.

Strengthening Exercise:

Strengthening of Muscles:

Enhancing the strength of the muscles around injured joints contributes to improved stability and support. This might be working with weight machines, free weights, or resistance bands while being supervised by a certified trainer or therapist.

Exercises using Isometry:

During isometric workouts, muscles are contracted without causing joint movement. Without placing undue pressure on the joints, these workouts aid in strength development. For knee osteoarthritis, for instance, static quadriceps contractions may be helpful.

Exercises For Range Of Motion And Flexibility:

Extending

Frequent stretches maintain or increase the range of motion in the injured joints and increase flexibility. Dynamic stretching may be especially helpful since it allows joints to move through their complete range of motion.

Tai Chi and Yoga:

These mindfulness exercises include deep breathing, meditation, and gentle movements. They may improve balance, flexibility, and general joint function, which makes them appropriate for managing osteoarthritis.

Techniques for Rehabilitation:

The use of heat and cold therapy

In order to reduce stiffness, heat treatment may assist in relaxing muscles and increase blood flow. Cold treatment has the ability to dull pain and reduce inflammation. It could be advised to switch between applications that are hot and cold.

Together Mobilization:

Manual methods are one way that physical therapists may mobilize and gently manipulate afflicted joints. This may lessen discomfort and increase joint mobility.

Helping Tools:

Braces are one kind of assistive device that may help afflicted joints by providing support. It's crucial to fit correctly and provide use instructions.

Education And Changing Your Way Of Living:

Education on body mechanics, lifestyle adjustments, and joint protection strategies should be a part of rehabilitation programs. This enables people to successfully manage their illness in day-to-day living.

In conclusion, a thorough approach to managing osteoarthritis with exercise and rehabilitation entails customizing programs to meet the needs of each individual, including low-impact exercises, placing a strong emphasis on strength training, encouraging flexibility, and using rehabilitation techniques under the supervision of medical professionals.

CHAPTER EIGHT

The Mind-Body Link In The Treatment Of Osteoarthritis

The treatment of osteoarthritis, a degenerative joint disease that predominantly damages joint cartilage, greatly benefits from an awareness of the mind-body link.

Including holistic methods that deal with osteoarthritis's psychological and physical components may help create a more thorough and successful treatment plan. Here's a detailed synopsis of the idea:

1. Handling Stress:

Stress may make osteoarthritis symptoms worse by causing inflammation and elevating pain thresholds. For those with osteoarthritis, putting stress management strategies into practice is essential. Stress reduction methods include gradual muscle relaxation, biofeedback, and deep breathing techniques. Reducing stress may have a beneficial effect on joint inflammation and pain perception, improving the quality of life for those with osteoarthritis in general.

2. Meditation & Mindfulness:

Being mindful entails focusing on the here and now without passing judgment. A crucial element of mindfulness is meditation, which promotes attentiveness and calm. Mindfulness may be very helpful in osteoarthritis in terms of pain management and general well-being enhancement. Programs for mindfulness-based stress reduction (MBSR), which often include meditation techniques, have shown promise in lowering pain and improving physical function in those with long-term pain issues, such as osteoarthritis.

3. Therapy Based On Cognitive Behavior (CBT):

The goal of cognitive behavioral therapy (CBT) is to alter maladaptive thinking and behavior patterns. CBT may assist people with osteoarthritis in learning coping mechanisms for pain management and adapting to the difficulties of having a chronic illness. Reducing maladaptive thinking patterns may help people feel less distressed about their discomfort and be better able to carry out everyday tasks.

4. Support Teams:

Enrolling in an osteoarthritis support group gives people the chance to interact with others going through similar struggles. Improving mental health may be facilitated by a supportive group where members share methods, coping mechanisms, and experiences. Support groups may also help people feel less alone and more a part of the community, which has a great impact on the psychological side of managing osteoarthritis.

5. Thinking Positively:

Keeping an optimistic mindset may have a big influence on how people see and treat their osteoarthritis. Thinking positively does not mean dismissing difficulties; rather, it means emphasizing one's capacity for adaptation and problem-solving. Optimism-building practices may enhance mental health and even improve how effectively pain is perceived.

In managing osteoarthritis, the mind-body link highlights the relationship between physical symptoms and psychological health. The holistic approach to controlling osteoarthritis may be strengthened by including stress management, mindfulness, cognitive behavioral therapy, support groups, and positive thinking in the entire treatment strategy.

People with osteoarthritis may enhance their overall well-being and quality of life by attending to both the physical and emotional components of the condition.

CHAPTER NINE
Using Technology To Improve Osteoarthritis Treatment

The common joint condition known as osteoarthritis (OA) is characterized by the deterioration of the underlying bone and cartilage. Since OA is a chronic ailment, managing it calls for an all-encompassing and dynamic strategy.

Technology integration has emerged as a possible way to optimize treatment techniques, improve patient outcomes, and increase access to healthcare for those with osteoarthritis. We will examine the function of many technology interventions in this streamlined solution approach, such as wearables, telemedicine, health apps, AI in treatment planning, and the next technological developments.

1. Wearable Technology:

The way medical professionals monitor and treat osteoarthritis has been completely transformed by wearable technology. These gadgets, which include activity trackers and smart watches, may record data in real-time about a patient's joint motions, sleep habits, and physical activity.

Wearables provide people with OA important insights into their everyday activities, which aid medical experts in customizing treatment strategies based on factual information. Because of this combination, early intervention and individualized treatment are made possible by OA management that is proactive in nature.

2. Telemedicine:

Access to healthcare may be facilitated in large part via telemedicine, especially for those with osteoarthritis and restricted mobility. There is less need for in-person visits when patients can communicate with medical providers virtually from the comfort of their homes. This method encourages prompt actions, improves care continuity, and makes remote monitoring easier. By offering instructional materials and encouraging self-management abilities, telemedicine also gives patients greater control over their treatment, which helps to promote a more patient-centered approach to osteoarthritis.

3. Apps For Health:

Osteoarthritis-specific health applications enable patients to take an active role in their care. These applications often come with features like the ability to monitor symptoms, remind you when to take your medications, and provide joint-healthy workout regimens. Health applications serve as a conduit for information sharing and communication between patients and healthcare professionals by using the capabilities of smartphones. These applications may also help with lifestyle adjustments like controlling weight and eating differently, which are important parts of treating osteoarthritis symptoms.

4. AI In The Planning Of Treatments:

Considerable progress is being made by artificial intelligence (AI) in the area of customized osteoarthritis therapy planning. Large-scale datasets including patient demographics, genetic data, and treatment results may be analyzed by machine learning algorithms to find trends and forecast the course of diseases. AI-powered solutions improve the efficacy of treatments by helping medical practitioners create customized treatment regimens based on unique patient features. Patients with osteoarthritis may get more accurate and focused therapy thanks to this data-driven approach.

5. Upcoming Developments In Technology:

Looking forward, a number of encouraging technical developments might further revolutionize the treatment of osteoarthritis:

Robotics in Rehabilitation: By offering precise and regulated motions to enhance joint function, robotic equipment may help with rehabilitation activities.

Augmented Reality (AR): By providing novel means of seeing joint anatomy and directing surgical procedures, AR apps may improve the accuracy of treating osteoarthritis (OA).

Genomic Medicine: New insights into the genetic variables impacting osteoarthritis susceptibility and development may be gained via advances in genomics, which will open the door to more individualized therapies.

Biosensors: Implantable biosensors may allow for ongoing joint health monitoring, providing real-time data for the early identification of changes in the state of the illness.

To sum up, using technology in the treatment of osteoarthritis is a revolutionary way to improve patient outcomes and expedite the provision of healthcare.

Together, these technological advancements—which range from telemedicine and wearable technology to AI-driven treatment planning and emerging trends—lead to a more thorough and patient-centered approach to controlling osteoarthritis. The opportunities to enhance the quality of life for those with osteoarthritis will increase as technology develops further.

Conclusion

In summary, the multimodal strategy of the simple solution approach to osteoarthritis aims to improve joint function, manage symptoms, and improve overall quality of life. Through comprehension of the essential ideas mentioned in the preceding sections, people may set off on a path to enhanced joint health and a higher standard of living.

Summary Of Main Ideas:

It's important to understand that osteoarthritis is a degenerative joint condition that causes pain, stiffness, and limited mobility due to the destruction of cartilage. Effective treatment begins with an understanding of the elements, such as age, heredity, and joint usage, that contribute to its development.

Modifications to Lifestyle: A key component of the Simplified Solution Approach is the modification of lifestyle. The key to controlling osteoarthritis is to maintain a healthy weight to minimize stress on joints, engage in joint-friendly activity, and eat a balanced diet full of nutrients that promote joint health.

Exercise and Physical Exercise: Osteoarthritis management requires regular physical exercise. Low-impact workouts that strengthen the muscles around joints, such as walking, cycling, and swimming, may aid. Individualized physical therapy regimens may improve joint function and reduce discomfort even further.

Medication Management: It's critical to collaborate closely with medical specialists to identify the right drugs for reducing pain and inflammation. Depending on how severe the symptoms are, doctors may give analgesics, DMARDs (disease-modifying antirheumatic medications), and non-steroidal anti-inflammatory medicines (NSAIDs).

Complementary treatments: Acupuncture, massage, and topical cream application are examples of complementary treatments that may provide further alleviation. These methods provide a comprehensive and individualized approach to managing osteoarthritis when paired with traditional therapies.

Joint Protection procedures: By being knowledgeable about and putting these procedures into practice, injured joints might avoid suffering further harm. This involves maintaining good posture, adjusting daily activities to lessen joint stress, and using assistive aids.

Motivation For Continued Self-Care:

One important and continuous part of controlling osteoarthritis is self-care. People are inspired to actively participate in their own well-being by:

Frequent Monitoring: It's critical to keep an eye on symptoms at all times and to take quick action in the event of any changes or flare-ups. This proactive strategy aids in making necessary adjustments to treatment regimens.

Open Lines of Communication with Healthcare Professionals: Having direct, honest lines of communication with healthcare professionals guarantees that any issues or queries will be answered right away. Frequent check-ups make it possible to assess the efficacy of therapy and make any required modifications.

Adopting Adaptive Strategies: Adopting joint-friendly behaviors, using ergonomic equipment, and changing activities may all improve long-term joint health and lessen the effects of osteoarthritis on day-to-day activities.

Mental and Emotional Health: It's critical to understand how osteoarthritis affects a person's mental health. A higher quality of life is often attained by partaking in activities that enhance mental and emotional health, such as mindfulness exercises, attending support groups, and keeping an optimistic mindset.

People with osteoarthritis may manage the condition's problems and enjoy active, satisfying lives by using this all-encompassing and customized strategy. Together, lifestyle changes, continuous self-care, and pharmacological treatments enable people to take control of their health and maximize their path to joint wellness.

THE END